The Aim of This Book,

The ghosts are in the negative attitude belonging in the Victorian era –

The human attitude towards female menopause in the 21st Century needs to change...

Females should no longer

'be seen and not heard!'

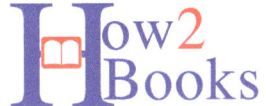

OUR PUBERTY BOOKS

For 9-11 and 11-14- & -18-year-olds...

Changes Facing Rosie & Changes Facing Kian 9-11 years

Changes Facing Caitlin & Changes Facing Jai 11-14- & 18-year-old teens

Do you have concerns?
Is your child entering puberty?

Please see

HORMONES, PUBERTY & YOUR CHILD
www.how2books.com.au

If you have purchased this book without its cover, it may be a stolen book.

Neither the publisher or the author is under any obligation to provide professional services in anyway, legal, health or in any form which is related to this book, its contents advice or otherwise.

The law and practices vary from country to country and state to state.

If legal or professional information is required, the purchaser, or the reader should seek the information privately and best suited to their particular needs, and circumstances.

This is not a medical book. It is a book developed by the publisher to open the conversation about how the human body changes when going into and through menopause.

The author and publisher specifically disclaim any liability that may be incurred from the information within this book.
All rights reserved. No part of this book, including the interior design, images, cover design, diagrams, or any intellectual property (IP), icons and photographs may be reproduced or transmitted in any form by any means (electronic, photocopying, recording or otherwise) without the prior permission of the publisher. ©

Copyright© 2023 MSI Australia
All rights reserved.

ISBN: 978-0-6457284-4-6

Published by How2Books
Under licence from MSI Ltd, Australia
Company Registration No: 96963518255
NSW, Australia

See our website: www.how2books.com.au
Or contact by email: sales@how2books.com.au
Covers and Copyright owned by MSI, Australia

MSI acknowledges the author and images, text and photographs used in this book.

WHY SHOULD THE SUBJECT OF MENOPAUSE BE HIDDEN?

Surely, from the time when women could not show their ankles in the Victorian era, many of these attitudes have come through to the generations now in the 21st Century

It is now time to change.

The human body is the human body, and the human brain is the human brain, the process of naturally changing times within all humans needs to be spoken about and the Victorian shroud needs to be removed from the human collective attitude!

CONTENT PAGE

CHAPTER ONE   1
GETTING TO THIS POINT

CHAPTER TWO   23
HORMONES, MENOPAUSE –
THE JOURNEY

CHAPTER THREE   40
AND WHAT HORMONE IS THAT?
THE 'HOW?' AND THE 'WHY?'

CHAPTER FOUR   68
PREMATURE-MENOPAUSE,
PERIMENOPAUSE, MENOPAUSE AND
POST-MENOPAUSE...

CHAPTER FIVE   88
STILL WANTING TO KNOW MORE...

CHAPTER SIX   106
CASE STUDIES -THE REALITY

INTRODUCTION

For generations females have suffered, not only with the Victorian attitude towards their sexuality, but towards the attitudes that women are a lesser human being than the males of the human species.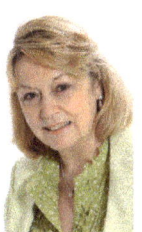

Testosterone plays a part in this, but more so does the attitude adopted by many males within the world populations. Many males, and indeed, some females who develop the attitude, 'they are more dominant' than their sister counterparts, may also relate to the role male dominance plays in society.

Biological females are born with great strengths in their mind and body. The distribution of strength is different to that of biological males, but none-the-less, it is a strength that has kept the human population moving forward for the last three hundred thousand years or since the time we evolved as homo-sapiens and came out of Africa.

Like the humans who live today, these ancient people would have liked to know, they can eat, rest, and enjoy their daily lives. Over this time these people evolved behaviours that helped them respond to the changes that happen within unstable environments.

We cannot dispute, the now collected scientific research, that proves the evolution of the species.

The ancient people, though we are now 'better educated,' we may think, also had working brains!

Through our development, and over time, males and females have developed larger brains; the hormones that worked in the bodies and brains of those earlier people, are inherited, and still working in our bodies and brains today. The earlier people had sex, made love, loved their families, and developed their attitudes.

So much of the working body are ancient without

modification. Some of the human brain has modified, but the hormones, enzymes and other bodily parts that allow us to survive and live our daily lives relate to the ancient and past generations!

When we take a deep breath and look back to the past, to our previous grandparents and past generations in our family line, we can see the ancient connections working inside our body and brain, and this is why, the actions, words said, and the attitudes, that belong in the past, need to be modernized.

Negative attitudes towards women, in the 21st Century are out of date. If these words are hitting home, that is a good sign you are sensitive to the meaning written in the above!

Christine

THE BRAIN IS CALLING

It was about 2am you know, and as I got up, the brain is still on the go…..!

Having just written four books on puberty for our teens as we know….!

There's another book to write, no time to rest, *'just take this name down the inner voice'* says….

'The Ghost of Female Menopause,' it speaks loudly for words I did not want to hear….

But, with a duty, I do as I'm told….
For writing about such subjects, one must surely be bold…!

Having written about hormones and the roles they play in our young people's lives; they venture to gain….

Many life experiences that are not always healthy, but they must try just to make their choices…!

For without some guidance, they don't have voices…

And so, it is, for women we know, who did not mention the struggle of menopause but still had a go….!

Many sad stories are told, how women managed through life's difficult times, and they still did not know…!

For we have technology, that helps us unfold, the journey of menopause and how it takes hold…!

Changes are made to our body and brain, and some of the actions we take are hard to refrain…

We don't know why we do what we do, but for some unknown reason, the deed is now done…!

Maybe, because all that was accomplished could so easily be undone…

A time of giving and having the kids, and what a struggle it had been…!

For little of the effort could be seen…..!

And yet, the memories are there, and the love of our children will help us get through –
for once menopause has passed, there's a starting and new…!

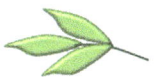

PREFACE

Oh, my gosh, and the fingers still want to push the keys on the keyboard, there is so much to do!

Yes, I have just finished writing the four-book series, 'Changes' on how our young adults, once they enter the pubertal years, how their body and brain change as they enter adulthood.

Like so much information about the human body and how it changes; this includes puberty, or any information related to human genitalia, it is still shrouded in old-fashioned, Victorian attitudes and the subject is too, 'pushed under the carpet,' and this is why so many young people, especially males, get into trouble, both within their communities and within the law.

Having taught and counselled young males at Huntercombe, Remand Centre, in Oxfordshire, United Kingdom, those young men taught me so much about the lack of pubertal education that has urged me to continue my work, and now onto menopause.

Have you ever taken a moment to look at the spelling and pronunciation of the word: <u>men o pause?</u> Surely, it implies that women are no longer enjoying sexual activities or indeed, enjoying being a woman…!

Aristotle, is one of the first philosophers to identify menopause, '*a time of change when a woman stops breeding…!*' In the 1930s menopause was described as a deficiency; this diagnosis led to many replenishment remedies being prescribed by medical practitioners, the prescriptions included, the crushed ovaries of many animals, also prescribed was testicular juice…!

As I do my research for this book, there still seems to be conflict and a lack of understanding in the research being undertaken by many foundations into the effects of menopause and the outcomes on the maturing population of females.

Not being in the research laboratory while writing this book, in some instances, I am using case studies of the experience's women have gone through to highlight the need for more understanding of the processes of menopause and why, in the 21st Century, half of the world population have either gone through menopause, or, are going through menopause, or will go through menopause later in life!

My research over a two-year period for the young adult books, 'Changes' has highlighted the role that hormones play in our body, not only in the way our body functions but also in the behaviour exhibited as our body, and brains go through the stages and processes needed to go through as we grow and mature.

CHAPTER ONE
GETTING TO THIS POINT

While writing, I have continued to teach and give public talks. My key area of teaching is psychology. Psychology is a great platform to work from, after all, psychology is the study of human behaviour. When we experience bodily changes, in many instances, our behaviours also change!

Throughout the dual career, as mentioned in the Preface, I have recently finished writing four books on puberty for young adults, and a support book for parents on the same subject. Whilst undertaking the research for the books, it gave me the perfect opportunity to develop the online education packages for schools on the subject. The young adult books are: 'Changes, Facing Rosie,' 'Changes Facing Kian,' 'Changes Facing Caitlin' and 'Changes Facing Jai', then to further write the supporting parents' book, 'Hormones, Puberty & Your Child,' after such writings and research, it was only natural that the follow-up book be on menopause.

This book is a natural progression, written in everyday language to support and help people who want to know more about how their body works and why at different times in life, we experience different bodily changes, and possibly different behaviours, even to the point that we revalue different uses of our time, thus, we start to think differently. As with the teen books, we need to start at the beginning, for without having a beginning, nothing on this planet of ours would happen!

Each of us, regardless of the life status we are born into, are created in the same way. Each of us, though we may have different coloured skin, eyes, hair, mannerisms, cultures, belief systems, habits, and values, we are all very similar on the inside! We each have a heart, lungs, brain, and other bodily parts that make us a biological male or female. I know there are differences, but this is not the intention of this book, this book is about the natural progression a biological woman's body takes as she progresses through life.

Of course, nothing is straight forward, we each have our journey, some easier than others, but none-the-less, it is still a journey!

THE BABY
When a baby girl is born, she is born with her eggs in place within her ovaries. A male baby will not make sperm until, as a child, the onset of puberty. Puberty, science is telling us, depending on heritage or ethnicity, we now know can start in some children as early as six to seven years of age, this of course has many variables and does not necessarily relate to all children of any group, but early puberty onset does happen!

The recognized age is about eight years old. When puberty starts, it is the movement of the sex hormones testosterone in males and estrogen in females that makes it happen. Hormones work on each person's individual body clock and each body clock works to its own body's rhythm!

In females, at puberty, the ovaries, adrenal glands, and the body's fat tissue produce estrogen. Both males and females create estrogen, but females create more. Estrogen helps the female body parts to function, including ovaries, vagina, breasts, and uterus. Now let's take one at a time.

OVARIES
Are the organs where the female eggs are stored. Though, females are born with their eggs in place, the eggs need to be stimulated and productive, and this starts as puberty slowly establishes itself in our young females. Estrogen supports the egg to grow and mature, and to become the ovum. The ovum, once mature, has the strength to travel through the fallopian tube.

At menopause, because of possibly low estrogen levels, the eggs have been discharged and the female is no longer fertile.

It is the changing estrogen levels that bring about, not only puberty, but also menopause!

VAGINA

Is the female body part that allows for intercourse to take place, and the blood from the menstruation, (period), formed in the uterus, to flow. Estrogen helps in vaginal health and wellbeing. It helps to support and promotes friendly flora to thrive and a healthy vaginal coating to be maintained. During menopause, the estrogen level may reduce leading to dryness and itching of the vaginal area!

UTERUS

Like so many areas of the body, the uterus needs to be supported and well looked after. Estrogen is responsible for keeping the mucus membrane, that lines the uterus, which keeps it in good order. It regulates the thickness and uterine mucus discharge, all of which help to support the healthy flora within the female body. The lack of estrogen being produced during menopause may result in the thinning of the uterus wall and lining.

BREASTS

Both males and females form breasts, but female breasts have the purpose, if a female wishes to feed a baby, she can do so. Female breast development happens because of estrogen and the role it plays in keeping the female body healthy and functional. Estrogen also plays a role in weaning by stopping the flow of milk when wanting to end breast feeding.

ESTROGEN

Like so many hormones, and as we journey through life, estrogen can fluctuate. I will continue to speak of '...*a healthy diet promotes healthy hormones...!*'

In some instances, not necessarily brought on by our environment or through lifestyle, hormones can and do change, and we may not know the reason!

Estrogen levels do vary and can fluctuate through and during menstrual cycles, pregnancy, strenuous exercise, weight gain, when using different or certain medications, drug taking, including recreational drugs, extreme, or spasmodic dieting, taking of some medications, primary ovarian insufficiency (Sometimes called premature ovarian failure), and other lifestyle changes.[1]

Contributing to low estrogen levels may be a congenital condition. If you have concerns, please contact your health professional.

THE FEMALE BABY

Part of the realization of teaching young adults about how their body functions and works, I take them back to the time of their conception. Because I directly relate to their own being and the time of their beginning, all children take a connected interest in how they started

---

[1] When the ovaries stop functioning, (about the age of 40), the release of eggs from the ovaries may become irregular. Estrogen is produced in the ovaries this may become irregular.

life. I then explain to the children about the fact, that all embryos start life as females. Boys find this difficult to accept! I then enlighten, '...*it is the development of the 'Y' chromosome at about eight weeks into the pregnancy that creates boys...!*'

When talking about girls, I clarify, '*At the time of her arrival, a baby girl's vagina is about one to two centimeters in length, so very tiny!*' I then continue, including both boys and girls, '...*at the time of your birth, all of your genital areas as babies are in miniature...!*' Because of the size, it does not mean that hormones are not working in their body! When a baby boy his born, his testosterone level is as high as that of a fourteen-year-old male teen.

As I continue my outline to the children, I explain many details, that all connect back to them.

I explain, '*To begin, the female egg, once mature, leaves the ovary and travels through the fallopian tube, the egg at this point is called an ovum. The female egg is the largest cell, and the male sperm is the smallest cell in our human bodies!'* When the children hear this, they always make a comment...

I give the children the information, by doing this, it helps to prevent any made-up stories about how their body is developing during puberty. They know the reasons of 'How?' and 'Why?' This information breaks down many barriers and helps in healthy discussion about their wellbeing.

To continue, *'if the egg (ovum) is not intercepted by a male sperm in the fallopian tube, the egg will reach the neck of the uterus. On doing this, the walls of the uterus, now a thick lining of blood, will be released, thus forming a period. A period can last between twenty-one to thirty-five days.'*

It is the healthy working hormones that allow the female body parts to work, and this is why we need to know the story from the beginning.

The hormonal system, also known as the endocrine

system, combines your body's organs and glands. Scientists have discovered over fifty hormones, there may be more, and yet, still waiting for discovery!

THE FEMALE BODY

Not spoken about to the children are the other parts of the female body. I concentrate on the natural processes both the male and female go through when hormones are activated as they journey into and through puberty!

However, in this book, I am going to speak about the clitoris and orgasm, both of which are part of the adult female body and behaviour.

It takes many hormones to keep the clitoris active and working in good order. The clitoris is equivalent to the male penis and should be included in adult conversations. It is a natural and essential part of the female body; the good working of this organ allows a woman to feel she is a woman!

Researchers and science have not understood how and why the clitoris has a role in the female body, they may ask, 'what is it's practical role?' or 'does it have a function other than that of female pleasure?' These questions have still not been answered!

There are three areas to the female clitoris, these are:

- ✓ <u>The crura</u>, there are two, and resemble a bracket like shape, these run from the glans (the head of the clitoris on the outside of the female body). The crura extend from the glans clitoris on the inside and on both sides within the tissue of the vulva.
- ✓ <u>The glans</u> is the visible part of the clitoris and is about one fifth of the size of the organ seen.
- ✓ <u>The bulbs and vestibule</u>, there is ongoing debate considering the bulbs or the vestibule.[2]

---

[2] Research, Dr. Helen O'Connell, Vincenzo, and Giulia Puppo
Five things you should know about the clitoris (medicalnewstoday.com)

These sections are identified as running either side of the vagina, thus, making up the whole section relating to the clitoris. The clitoris may extend to seven centimeters in length and into the female body.

The sexual health of females needs to be considered not only in younger women but in women who are going through, perimenopause and or through menopause.

As the mature woman's body is mature, the body does not lose its functions and desire for intercourse and the enjoyment of sex and love.

Women who have gone through menopause still have sexual feelings and desires. It is not wrong for a woman to satisfy her own sexual needs, which in return add to her own mental, physical wellbeing and good health.

The human body, both male and female, has needs, and personal sexual gratification relieves tension, may release headaches caused through stress, and can help to re-balance the body's natural rhythms.

THE BODY'S ELECTRONICS

The male penis, female vagina, and clitoris have, like so many areas of the body and brain, an electrical system that is connected to the brain, through neuron pathways that run throughout the body. The genital electronics, in both males and females are known as 'free' nerve endings. In both the male penis, female clitoris and vagina, this free nerve ending allows for sexual satisfaction and intense sensations that may lead to orgasm in females and ejaculation in males.

It is the stimulation from either the enjoyment of sex before and after menopause that keeps the female genitalia active and in good health.

Stimulation, through sexual activity or through the body being touched and loved, allows, through the electronic connections, to the senses, which then stimulates the hormones to become active in the genitals of both females and males. It is the release of hormones that keeps the vagina clean and healthy, the wholeness of the woman from the inside, the positive self-esteem, the maintenance of libido, the gratification of self and the enjoyment of life.

Having said all the above, the clitoris is still taboo if spoken about in public places, and yet, it is as much a part of the female's body as the vagina, breasts, brain, nose, or lips on her face, or for the mention of the male penis...! It is the attitude still connected to the Victorian era, that limits conversation when speaking of the male and female genitalia.

Again, I have mentioned hormones, hormones are the vehicles that allow both males and females to go into puberty, and in females into menopause.

SEVERAL GLANDS MAKE UP THE HORMONES IN YOUR BODY AND BRAIN

PINEAL, the pineal gland which sits in the middle of your mid-brain. This gland is possibly the least understood of the endocrine system. Science tells us that it helps to control melatonin levels, which are part of your sleep patterns, they are otherwise known as the circadian rhythms. During both puberty and menopause, there seems to be a disconnect with the melatonin hormone. Many teens find it difficult to sleep as do many women going through menopause.

HYPOTHALAMUS, the hypothalamus gland, is found towards the base of the brain, and is above the pituitary gland. Its role is important as it has a direct link between the endocrine and nervous system of your body and brain.

THYROID, the gland sits in your neck and resembles the shape of a butterfly. This gland produces and secretes different hormones essential to health and wellbeing.

PARATHYROID, this gland is attached to the back of the thyroid gland. The parathyroid gland plays an important role in balancing both the phosphorus and calcium in your blood and bones.

ADRENAL, glands are often referred to as releasing the 'fight or flight' hormone adrenaline; these glands sit on top of your kidney which are in the lower part of your back.

PANCREAS, releases insulin which controls the sugar or glucose levels in your blood supply. In diabetes type one, children, and adults, diagnosed with diabetes, no longer produce insulin. If insulin is produced, it may be in minimum quantities which does not allow for the control of sugar levels entering the blood stream.

OVARIES, produces some estrogen and the associated estrogen hormones including estradiol, estriol and estrone.

- **Estrogen** helps to make your bones stronger and helps to keep the heart and brain healthy.

- **Estradiol** levels can vary depending on the phase of the female menstrual cycle. It is also involved with the adjustment of the female reproductive cycles. During puberty it supports the development of breasts, widening of the hips and the fat distribution within the body.

- **Estriol**, like estrone, and estradiol, helps the female body to grow and become ready for womanhood.

- **Estrone** can store estrogen and helps with female development and plays a part in female reproductive health. Like most hormones, these work with your body's clock.

TESTES are in the male scrotum. Testes produce testosterone and like so many hormones, females also produce smaller amounts of testosterone which helps to balance estrogen levels.

The above-mentioned are just the start; the subject of identifying how the endocrine system works takes many years of professional and medical study, all too much in a short book of this nature.

Most women reading this book are possibly looking for answers to their changing conditions or condition as they enter menopause. However, without an understanding of how the body and endocrine system works, it's difficult to start on the journey of change...!

THE GIFT – THE WOMAN'S BODY

A female I was born,
at the time, I didn't have a say…!

But you know what, I was glad I was born this way…!

Through puberty I grew, and then, and if only I knew…

Breasts would grow; size was of no concern, for they had a purpose and nature knew best….

For time would tell, then I'd find out the rest…!

A mother I become, when first, I produced a son…!

Life has its moments, as most mums know… and as we watch our children grow…

For none of this would be possible if a girl was not born…

Later to become a mother and a body to love, had this have not happened, nor would any of the above……………!

LOVE BEING A WOMAN

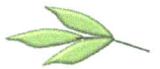

Taking the mystery out of how the human body works allows us to learn how to work with our body through different and changing times in life.

Having such information reduces stress, allows us to find answers to worrisome question, and benefits our health and wellbeing.

Menopause may be the end of a woman's reproductive years, but it can be a time of ultimate growth for the female.

By using our time responsibly, creating 'moments in time' each female can grow in her heart, mind, and soul!

It is indeed a time for growth and developing long awaited dreams.

YOUR NOTES

CHAPTER TWO
HORMONES, PERIMENOPAUSE OR MENOPAUSE – THE ENDOCRINE SYSTEM – THE JOURNEY...!

While undertaking the research and writing of the children's books, it is only natural, and with thought, that the journey of our hormones should include, menopause, a time of chemical changes within the female body and brain.

Just to mention, there is a conversation within our communities that also have the idea, that many males go through puberty. Many males may experience fewer erections, because of a lower testosterone output, but it is not the menopause that females go through. I will concentrate on females as the changes to the female body and brain, can in some instances, alter the very pathway and progression of their lives.

I'm including the brain, as many educators, and indeed, independent medical professionals often relate hormone changes to just the body, when in fact, hormone changes include the whole of the human being, including the way they think and behave, and both thinking and behaving include the working brain!

As I delved deeply into the role hormones play in our lives, it started to answer many questions to the, sometimes, bizarre behaviour we can independently display at different times as we go through the bodily and brain changes necessary to equip us females for the next journey of our lives.

The chemical structure of hormones varies with different experiences we endure or are exposed to. I have been through menopause at the age of forty-four. I had no idea of what was going on in my body, and indeed my head! Like so many women, I was prescribed hormone replacement therapy or HRT, and quickly, after a month or two, decided that the therapy was not for me, and would let nature run its course. I cannot say if it was a good or bad decision, but that was my choice! When medical practitioners, speak to their patients, they might say, '*It is the reduced levels of estrogen, that bring about menopause….!*' Technically, that is correct. But, having experienced, my own experiences of menopause, I now believe there are many variations of perimenopause, menopause, and post menopause!

My next awareness of hormones came about while I was researching the facts on food additives for my book, *'Devils In Our Food'*. Please let me expand here, at the age of ten years, our beautiful child was diagnosed with juvenile onset diabetes or (diabetes type one). The hospital we attended for the condition, offered many educational packages, which, I watched and learnt from.

I exhausted the hospital's resources, but still wanted to know more! From the educational experience that remains in my mind, it is the role of complex carbohydrates and carbohydrates. This knowledge also helped me when writing the *'Devils In Our Food'* book, and when writing and recording other programs that relate to our food and the impact poisons have on the human body and system. To that point, some of the food chemicals now going into food and drink alter children and adult behaviour; different behaviour is brought about by the messages sent from the brain which can reinforce different, in many instances, negative behaviours, words spoken, and acts committed!

Before negative behaviours take place, the hormone supply to the brain of a perpetrator must alter, this may be done through the hormones, (chemical messengers), being altered through either poisonous or dangerous substances within drugs or substances taken or by the food or drink being ingested!

Further reinforcement of the role hormones plays in our body and brain came about as I researched the information for the children's books mentioned in chapter one. Over the last four-five years, I spent three years teaching sex (pubertal) education. I knew that something was missing in the information I was teaching and over a two-year period continued researching. Again, it was the hormone story. Yes, the children were learning about puberty and some of the facts, but they were not getting the whole story!

Having taught the subject, I knew there had to be a 'HOW?' and 'WHY?' to this topic within the information I was giving to the young teens. Most young people want to learn, and if the information is given in succinct facts, they can learn everything that comes their way. It is important that we learn to present to children and adults, whole stories and not just part of the picture, this is why the 'HOW?' and 'WHY?' are so important within any learning children, or, as adults, we do.

Now, back to my journey of menopause, and to the hormones that make menopause happen. My journey seemed to last just one to two months; it was abrupt and traumatizing to have such drastic change in such a short space of time, or was I in perimenopause? I know I had mood swings, violent pains coming from the ovary area of my body. I can remember, rolling around on the kitchen floor in agony with the pain. Slowly, after taking medication, the pain seemed to ease off. It was like a magnitude period pain, but no period at the time; that was to come later!

The menopause may have been longer, I know I suffered fierce headaches, aching limbs, all of which I now know are the signs of perimenopause, not only was the body under attack, but there were changes taking place in my attitude. The marriage had been difficult, but the children and home were always a priority. I am sure so many women can relate to this story. As women, we mainly put ourselves last, this is not always wise, but just the same, it is the love of the children and home that holds so many families together.

To verify the above, I had two little children at school, studying in post-graduate studies at university, and I was working in many part-time, public sector, short-term contracts. Sitting in an office one day, I was experiencing severe pains in my arms and body; I felt ghastly. I made an appointment with the doctor and on diagnosis, I had a type of glandular fever. The glandular fever led to a quick *'change of life'* in menopause happening in a hurry….!

As I have said, I was living in a difficult marriage, times had been tough, but like many females, especially those in many faith families, we are taught to 'put up and endure', that was the upbringing!

My experience of menopause or perimenopause had devastating outcomes. Eventually, the marriage was no more!
In the fifties and sixties, couples, they may have had sex before marriage, but it was never spoken

about, nor was the fact of puberty, menopause, and the like life changes we may experience! For public view, sex was to wait until the wedding day and not a day sooner! Had single women decided to co-habitat with a male, the degrading and derogatory names and others would be said, mainly in gossip, while hanging out the washing or while the next-door neighbour hangs over the fence while drinking their cup of tea! Consequently, these attitudes allowed many couples to commit to marriage without the woman or man knowing much about the other! More directly, the habits and behaviours they had and the living environment they created. It is with such living environments, when a woman experiences changes such as menopause, they too, start to re-evaluate their life direction and living conditions!

CHANGING ATTITUDES

Going back to the fifties and sixties, the remnants of the Victorian era and into the 21st Century, are still hanging in people's attitudes; change is difficult when it is the attitude of millions of people that needs to change.

Such were the attitudes our parents had, these handed down from their parents and grandparents…! On occasion, I now laugh to myself. As a child, I would often hear commented from neighbours and sometimes family members, '*She/he, has had a nervous breakdown…!*' A nervous breakdown seemed to relate to anybody who was experiencing changes in their lives or was finding managing everyday life difficult! Thankfully, times have moved on a bit, and in some examples have changed, but sadly, not in many held attitudes, for the better in many instances.

Many women experience long-term menopausal change over a ten-year span. Many of these women live in misery and discomfort trying to manage their every day-to-day living, and like so many families, the family looks on, not understanding the 'HOW?' and 'WHY?'

As I journeyed on, I needed to know more, it led to more and more reading. Science is proving that hormone changes may happen in both the male and female body and brain through the actions we each take! Actions may include gambling, and other developed negative habits, diet, drug abuse and other actions detrimental to the wellbeing of the human body and brain! Surely, if hormones are altered, so must be the human body's endocrine system, after all, it is the story of the 'fuel in the tank!' If you develop destructive habits, put cheap, lousy food or drink in your Maserati, (your body), your beautiful car, is not going to run properly! Similarly, if you develop bad or negative habits, you will eventually pay the price! As I have said, to date, science is telling us that there are over fifty hormones within the human body and some of those fifty live in the brain. There may be more and as technology becomes advanced, more hormones may be found. Hormones, and as mentioned, are part of the working endocrine system. The endocrine system incorporates the supply of insulin to the body when extra insulin is required to stabilize excessive sugars. The endocrine system also supplies extra adrenaline when you need to run out of trouble or run or hide to keep yourself safe!

So, hormones play an essential role in your body and brain. Hormones allow us to think, laugh, play, and do the serious jobs needing to be done; they are after all, the chemical messengers connecting your brain and body together allowing you to work as one!

Because of varying hormone supplies during both puberty and menopause, many developed habits, such as eating over processed food, or drinking too much artificial soft drink, consuming too much alcohol, your digestive system may become sensitive to artificial foods and drinks, adding excess weight, or changing behaviour, not to mention, gut discomfort! Please remember, your bad habits interfere with your natural hormone supplies!

Numerous hormones work within different parts of the body and brain, and many work on their own time clocks as in the onset of puberty and menopause. Each person's body clock is programmed to work at different times in their lives.

I now believe that different body clocks can be re-programmed after different life-changing events we experience.

Since the onset of Covid in 2019, studies are now showing that there is an increase in children developing type one diabetes. This information was released from the Centres for Disease and Prevention, USA. The numbers of Australian children developing this condition is also reported to have increased during, and post Covid. We also need to be aware, will there be a rise in pre-menopausal or perimenopausal women since the Covid pandemic? More studies are needed to verify the findings. What we need to acknowledge, is that many conditions are brought on by the hormones in our bodies becoming disrupted by different environments and pathogens. If this is so with Covid, this may be the case with many other viruses that invade our bodies!

With advancing technology, and the knowledge that hormones play a critical role in everybody's day-to-day life, we need to expand and explain the information, not only to the adults of the world, but too, to our children and grandchildren.

The word menopause has not had public space or been in the community of global conversations, but this is now the opportunity for this subject to, not only be heard, but to be a GLOBAL headline.

DO NOT LINGER ON PAST EVENTS

When we hurt, it's hard to forget, and yet, for those times should not be….

Many women hide the hurt they feel, and try to move on, and have freedom of will….!

But the experience is indelible and etched in stone, for the memory is still…!

The abuse and hurt from it all, we want to forget and make as new, but the pain and memory will not go away….!

We pretend, and carry on, shopping to get, ironing to do, homework to help, cleaning right through…!

Regardless of experiences, the attitude persists, '…*make the most of it….,*' '…*you made your bed, now lie in it…*' they said…

And sometimes you think, 'I'd rather be dead…!'

No, '…*that is not the attitude…*' your inner voice says, past experiences can make you strong, and allow you to hear the hummingbird's song…

Keep going you must, for there is so much in the world that needs to be done…

For what you have learnt will release you from fear….

Making changes may be difficult to do, through tears and hurt, the learning is sent, not to mention the abuse without consent...!

The strength and the knowledge gained through such times, the remnant and seeds persist...

They only continue to hold while you allow and insist......!

LIFE IS FOR LIVING AND LEARNING

> *It's time to speak up and to speak loudly. Our parents and grandparents were gagged by old Victorian attitudes that have caused hurt, pain, and humiliation to many women; that needs to stop in the 21st Century...*

As each female goes through menopause, she may realize that life is too short to worry about trivia!

She may realize that she wants change in her life, in fact to grow and to complete her journey, she may embark and make that change happen...!

All people have a purpose, and it is a female's responsibility to find that purpose...!

CHAPTER THREE
AND WHAT HORMONE IS THAT?
THE 'HOW?' AND THE 'WHY?'

Our sex hormones take us into and through puberty, these same hormones want to retire once they have done their jobs through our fertility years, and like many areas of the human brain and body, there is a natural process in slowing down. Slowing down, however, doesn't mean STOP, it means take the time, have some fun and enjoy the moments in life. I love to have some fun when I write, and writing the teen books on puberty, 'Changes' allowed me to 'let my head go' and 'my hair down!'

And why should I not extend this fun to my adult readers, there is no reason why at all…?

Chapter one and two have been to the point, but now we all need a refreshing change, and change starts now.

While writing the young adult books, I came to a dilemma, and that was, 'how do I teach young adults about hormones, when they are a chemical structure and extremely boring to look at and learn?' While doodling, I came up with my solution, 'Hormones with Hats', and now let's move on to this fascinating area of this book. As I have said, 'hormones are chemical messengers,' and many work from the moment of conception, until death.

Hormones help to keep us healthy and allow us to live our daily lives. They are essential if the body is to perform different movements, make different choices and to let us know when to eat, drink, fight, or flight; they are an essential part of the living system in animals, insects, and human beings.

GROWTH HORMONE

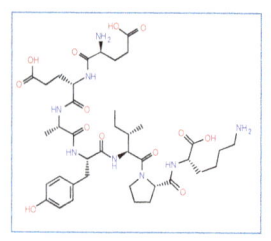

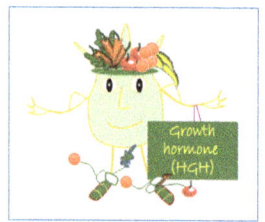

The growth hormone chemical, as seen opposite,[3] is the first in many chemicals, I would like to speak about in this section.

This hormone works at the very onset during your conception in the multiplying and division of cells to become an embryo, and then a baby. It works until we each take our last breath! Throughout life, and possibly a minor role, once we have stopped growing and developing, the growth hormone assists with hair and nail growth and possibly some other body repairs as in broken bones or surgery recovery.

Many hormones do not work alone, some rely on a support system and estrogen is one such hormone!

---

[3] Image courtesy: Human growth hormone (32-38) Structure - C39H60N8O13 | Mol-Instincts

ESTROGEN HORMONE

Estrogen is the name given to a group of hormone compounds. It is a main hormone and is essential to the menstrual cycle which can go from twenty-one to thirty-five days.

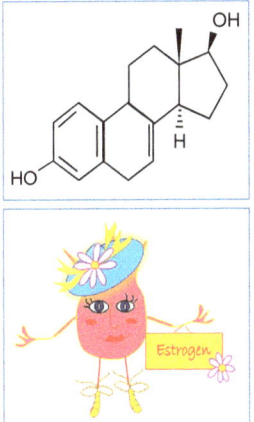

Estrogen helps a body to mature. It also helps to keep your bones strong, and to keep the heart and brain healthy.

Women have three types of hormones that work within the reproductive menstrual cycle: estrogen, estradiol and estriol.

Estrogen binds together estradiol and estriol. Both males and females have this hormone. In addition to regulating the menstrual cycle, estrogen affects the reproductive tract, urinary tract, heart, blood vessels, bones, breasts, skin, hair, mucous membranes, including those in the uterus and that which surrounds the mature ovum after leaving the ovary and entering the fallopian tube, pelvic muscles, and the brain. Secondary sexual characteristics, such as pubic and armpit hair, also start to grow when estrogen levels rise. Many organ systems, including muscles, skeletal and cardiovascular systems, and the brain are affected by the supply of estrogen.

ESTRONE HORMONE

Estrone can store estrogen and helps with female development and plays a part in female reproductive health. Like most hormones, these work with your body's clock. Many hormones can be sensitive to your body changes.

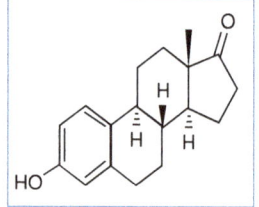
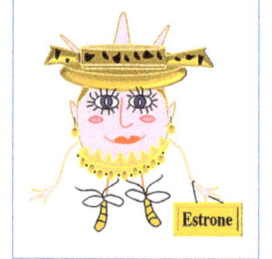

An example may be seen with severe dieting without medical advice or guidance.

Estrone can be synthesized from cholesterol and secreted from the gonads and from the body's fatty tissue. (Both males and females have gonads). Estrone is a weaker hormone than estrogen but can be converted, if needed, to estrogen by the body. It is good for,
- Bone health
- Cognitive function (your brain function) and
- The production of nitric oxide, a molecule that helps blood vessels open and function.

All the hormones spoken about so far, need to work in balance; for effective bodily functions (as previously mentioned), many hormones work with more than one hormone.

Your body, though you are living in the 21st Century, is an ancient system that has taken many thousands of years of evolution to make it what it is today. During puberty and menopause, more science is showing us, your body responds positively to the intake of whole food!

ESTRADIOL HORMONE

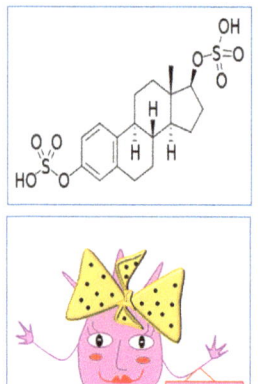

Estradiol is principally a female hormone, produced primarily in the female ovaries. The levels can vary depending on the phase of the female menstrual cycle. It is also involved with the adjustment of the female reproductive cycles.

It helps the female body in the maintenance of the reproductive tissue within the uterus and the breasts.

Estradiol helps maintain memory, increases sexual interest in males and females, improves mood and happiness and improves the quality of your sleep.

In Males, it regulates sex drive, it helps in achieving erections, the production of sperm and testicular function.

PROGESTERONE HORMONE

Progesterone is released from the female ovaries. It helps when females start to have their periods, and in the body's control of the menstrual cycle.

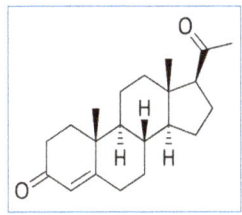

It, like many other hormones, has many functions. Before fertilization, it supports the function of human sperm in the migration through the female vaginal tract after intercourse.

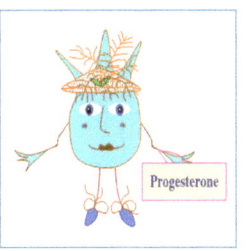

Progesterone plays a key role in breast development and supports the maturation of breasts (mammary glands), during pregnancy which allows for lactation to develop allowing the mother to breastfeed her infant.

In males, it is the precursor to testosterone production, it also helps to balance male estrogen.

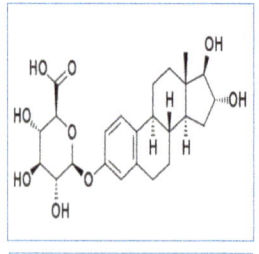

ESTRIOL HORMONE

Estriol, like estrone, and estradiol, helps the female body to grow and become ready for womanhood.

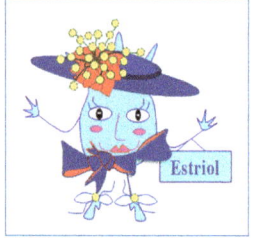

Like so many hormones, it too, works with its own clock and will click into gear when it receives certain messages from your brain.

Research is revealing, Estriol appears to offer a wide range of health benefits to several health conditions, some of which include rheumatoid arthritis, multiple sclerosis, thyroiditis, and psoriasis. Estriol is at its highest during pregnancy and at childbirth.

In males it is in the fatty tissue of the testicles, and brain.

TESTOSTERONE HORMONE

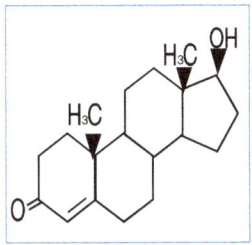

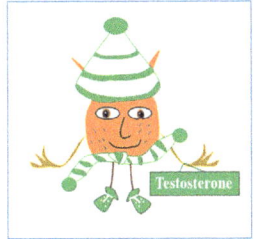

Testosterone is the key to males being males. It's the male sex hormone that controls their red blood cell production, muscle mass, fat distribution and fertility.

Females also produce testosterone, but at a much-reduced quantity.

In both males and females, testosterone helps with mood and feelings, cognitive or brain support with learning, remembering, planning and other necessary brain functions. It also supports bone and muscle health, and the development of body hair.

In females, testosterone is produced in the ovaries and adrenal glands. In males, it is produced in the testes and adrenal glands and is key to a healthy prostate gland. In both males and females, testosterone is an important hormone in both brain and heart health. In males, it plays a key role in reproduction. Low levels of testosterone have been attributed to food and drink additives, including soft drinks, coloring dyes, and other synthetic chemicals added to the world food supply chain.

GHRELIN HORMONE

Ghrelin is the hormone, (opposite [4]), that lets you know when you feel hungry. If people eat when they are not hungry, for instance, junk food can make you feel full and about an hour later after the meal, you feel hungry again!

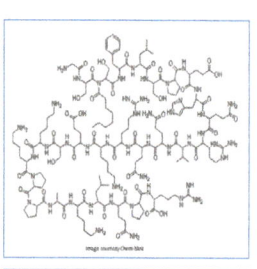

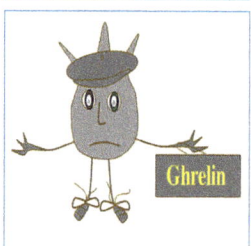

When this happens, your ghrelin hormone release may become confused. Your gut sends a message

---

[4] Image courtesy Chem Blanc

to your brain saying, '*I'm hungry.*' The message is received by the hypothalamus in the brain. The hormones: ghrelin is just one!

Hormones are sensitive triggers to your body's needs, and if the hormone and brain receive confused information, as in the eating of junk food and drink, then you may trigger an oversupply of ghrelin! Ghrelin's main function is to increase appetite and can encourage eating more food than is possibly necessary for a healthy body to function. Through both puberty and menopause, there may be a desire to eat, over fat, processed, over-processed sugary food; this desire should be avoided. If there are cravings, try a slice of whole meal bread with a light covering of natural honey; it works wonders.

The nature of the hormone may encourage eating more calorie foods, the energy from this food is stored in the body's fat, thus increasing weight if the extra calories are not used in work or exercise!

ADRENALINE HORMONE

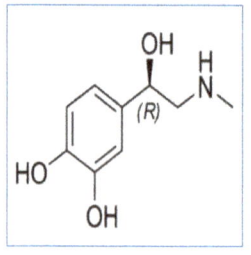

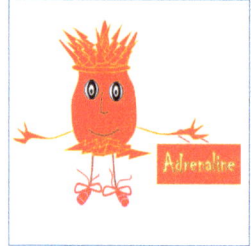

The adrenaline glands sit on top of the kidneys and work almost remotely until they are needed in an emergency or in times of facing different stress or stressors!

The adrenal hormone, gland is responsible for making many hormones, including, cortisol, aldosterone, adrenaline, and noradrenaline. The adrenaline gland is controlled by the pituitary gland in the brain.

As you may be aware, adrenaline is also known as the 'fight or flight' hormone, though helpful in times of stress, too much adrenalin can make you anxious, nervous, or excited, therefore it is important to manage adrenaline and the like hormones. Menopause can be a time of heightened anxiety, this may be the result of too much adrenaline, if so, go on regular walks, try to slow down by giving yourself valuable 'ME' time, practise deep breathing and other quality times that work for you.

It takes many healthy hormones to keep our body and brain working well.

It is the importance of the 'WHY?' and 'HOW?'

CORTISOL HORMONE

Cortisol is sometimes referred to as the stress hormone; it is a naturally occurring hormone which is made by the adrenal gland.

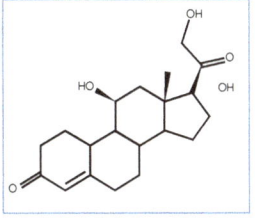

The hormone is used throughout the body which is controlled by the hypothalamus.

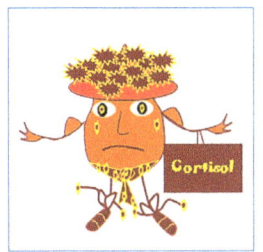

Most cells and cell receptors in the human body contain and work with cortisol. Cortisol is important to maintain your metabolism and/or sugar levels, lowering body inflammation, the salt and water balance of the body, memory formation, foetal development in the unborn child, and blood pressure. Cortisol also helps in the digestion of your food and manages how your body works to separate the protein, fat, or carbohydrate from the food eaten! This is why, when we feel stress, sometimes it is impossible to eat and sometimes, when in a stressful situation, we eat too much...!

It is important to keep cortisol levels manageable, this can be done again, through sport, exercise, meditation or breathing exercises.

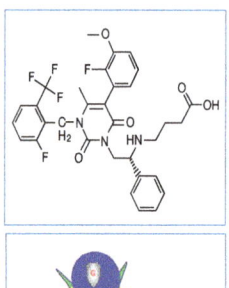

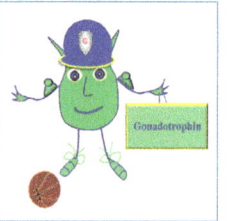

GONADOTROPIN HORMONE

The hormone Gonadotropin's main purpose is to help to control the functions within the ovaries and testes.

Gonadotropins are important for the regulation and proper

functioning related to male and female reproduction.

The main role of gonadotropin is to work with the gonads, meaning, the gonad is the sex reproductive gland in both males and females. Gonadotropins are made in the pituitary gland in response to other hormone stimulation in the hypothalamus in the brain. The process of production is carried out by the hypothalamus pituitary gonad axis. There are three areas of gonadotropins, which again consist of two peptide chains, keeping in mind, a peptide is smaller than a hormone, and in this instance, works to support both testosterone and estrogen.

As said, the gonads are the sex or reproductive glands in both females and males. The female reproductive cell are egg cells, and in males, the reproductive cells are sperm!'

SEROTONIN HORMONE

Serotonin helps with mood adjustment, developing regular sleep patterns, bone health, helps wounds or cut skin to heal, supports your digestive system.

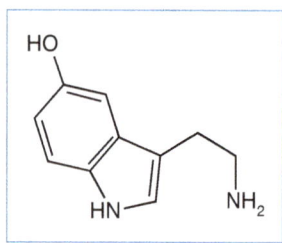

It helps with learning and academic attainment, but it too, helps with libido, or sexual drive, and desire.

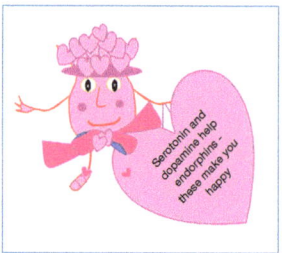

When serotonin is balanced and working in the human body, it also helps with 'happiness' feelings. When serotonin is not balanced, you will know by the feelings of sadness. When there is reduced serotonin, we can feel lonely or unhappy. Reduced serotonin can lead to problems in mental health, depression, anxiety, mood swings, suicidal behaviour, panic disorders, digestive, and sleep problems, phobias, and, or schizophrenia.

If, you have concerns over any of the above, please speak to your health professional.

To help maintain a balanced serotonin level, eat a healthy diet, do regular exercises, develop a project, and take the time to enjoy the moments.

We can all support the good health of our hormones by eating a balanced and healthy diet. Some suggested foods for serotonin balance, include salmon, eggs, cheese, turkey, pineapples, fresh nuts, oats, and seeds.

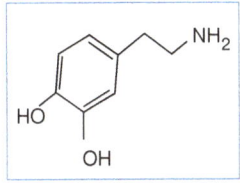
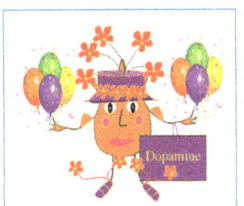

DOPAMINE HORMONE

When there are high levels of dopamine in the brain, you will want to 'party!' Continuous partying is not good for your health, brain, or learning new skills.

When dopamine becomes 'overcharged' – this happens in drug, alcohol, vaping or through other abuse substances, the brain creates a habit to 'party...!' Partying in older adults may include, alcohol abuse, gambling, including poker machines, smoking, self-neglect to feed the gambling habit, and other developed habits that are not conducive to your human wellbeing.

However, when dopamine is balanced, it helps with the following:

- ✓ focus and attention to different jobs.
- ✓ developing skills such as driving a car, and operating machinery.
- ✓ it helps and contributes to motivation, and to mood and regular sleep patterns.

Dopamine assists with control of nausea or vomiting and how we process pain. It assists with blood vessel and kidney function and body movement and assists with your heart rate. It also assists with memory function.

OXYTOCIN HORMONE

Oxytocin, or the 'love hormone' in so many instances is not understood! Many people experience different emotional states when they think they are in love! These states work with our emotions, which are connected to our hormone supply in our brain and other areas of our body. During our teen years, because of higher levels of hormones, it is possibly easier to think or fall in love than later in life!

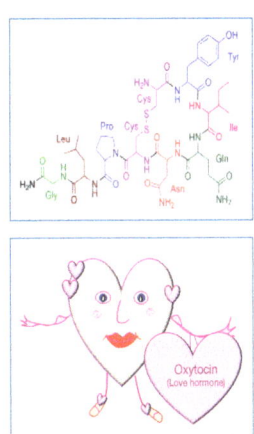

Many 'love' experiences can be painful, but they are 'life experiences!' When a person feels hurt through the experience of unrequited love, their oxytocin levels may reduce... This condition can lead to, stress, poor self-esteem, lack of sleeping properly, and lack of confidence.

It is not only the teens that are affected by low

levels of oxytocin, but it can also and does happen to older people. If you feel you may have low oxytocin levels, please seek medical support.

Other outcomes of low oxytocin levels may include limited touching, and feelings of abandonment. Remedies for this situation include,
- ✓ go out with other people, you don't have to be in love with a person to enjoy their company.
- ✓ hobbies and projects are great to have when life seems like hell on the other side of the front door!
- ✓ reconnect with old friends, and importantly, reconnect with family members.

DO NOT TAKE REVENGE IF YOU ARE HURT, BE CREATIVE AND FIND ANOTHER DIRECTION

MELATONIN HORMONE

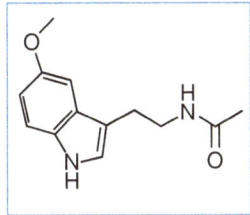

Melatonin is made in the pineal gland, a small pea-sized gland, found in the middle of the human mid-brain.

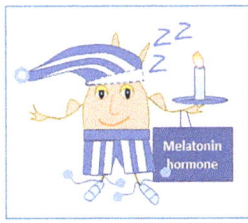

Melatonin works as a stimulant to the body and tells you when to sleep or when to wake up!

This hormone works in response to darkness. A normal melatonin level will support you to have a good night's sleep!

In reduced melatonin levels, often experienced with teens and when females start to go through menopause, it may cause mood swings, disruption in sleep pattens, depression and other health conditions.

Like so many hormones, this hormone too, works with your body clock and the forces of night and day. Once evening starts to descend, the body clock kicks in, when melatonin is balanced, you will start to feel sleepy.

Melatonin levels, in healthy people are elevated for around twelve hours, allowing people to work, study, play or do hobbies. With such activities in the day, a normal melatonin level will support people to have a good night's sleep! Melatonin has many roles, it not only regulates the sleep cycle, in females, it plays a role in the menstruation cycle.

However, too much melatonin can cause headaches, drowsiness, nausea, and dizziness.

Like all hormonal levels, each needs to be balanced in the body. By eating a balanced diet that is rich in, vegetables, comprising a variety of fruits, including bananas, berries, cherries, oranges, pineapple, corn, asparagus, tomatoes, olives, broccoli, peanuts, sunflower seeds, flaxseed, and mustard seeds also include in the diet, chicken, eggs, fish, cheese and some whole grain, complex carbohydrate, such as whole grain breads. All these foods help to increase your melatonin level.

HORMONES

So overlooked they seem to be, and yet, those little hormones work in our body and brain, and don't charge a fee….!

They have such a mighty job to do, and to make sure we respond and work right through…!

Some work through the night, others allow us to react, when we feel the fear and the fright…!

'Hormones With Hats', I mentioned one day… only to hear the people say,

'Hormones With Hats', that's a funny name, but much of a novelty, just the same…!

How else, I replied, can I make people aware of the importance of hormones, and without despair…!

When our hormones are healthy, we feel just great, no time to feel unhappy, no time to feel hate…!

So, you see, it's to your advantage to know, why these little hormones you know little about…

Are part of the chemistry, that keeps you safe and well, for without their work, you may feel like hell…!

So much is underestimated by the role that hormones play in the human body and brain. When our hormones are interrupted, we find it difficult to work, rest or play. A healthy diet will support hormone levels.

Leave out of your diet 'junk food' and anything that has artificial additives or preservatives!

As females enter this new phase of life, there's a certain awareness of their own independence; they may feel they want to achieve more or to be accomplished; there's sometimes a calling from within

It's time to listen to the inner voice...

It's time to make independent choices that allow for self-fulfilment in the actions you take and the accomplishment you make...

CHAPTER FOUR
PREMATURE MENOPAUSE, PERIMENOPAUSE, MENOPAUSE AND POST-MENOPAUSE...

Is it premature menopause? Some health professionals do not use this term. Perimenopause, menopause, and post-menopause are confusing terms when a woman is in the middle of 'change' in her life. As I continue to research on menopause, the medical information becomes ever more difficult to understand.

The medical community has informed information on menopause in medical journals, in researched papers, and in different medical apps on the worldwide web, but it does not always take this condition back to how people suffer in both their physical and mental health!

As I have mentioned in Chapter Two, I was told at forty-four years of age, *'You are premature menopausal!'* Putting this timing into perspective, this was over thirty years ago. I am now a grandmother and am still confused by my behaviour over that time. I had no idea of what premature menopausal meant, and I'm still slightly confused! The menopause, a time of change within everywoman's life happens, in some young women, when they are in their twenties!

There has been a shroud of silence, I see it as the Victorian attitude, that has been handed down from generation to generation. The attitude of *'being seen and not heard,'* doesn't only apply to women going through menopause, but also to children and young adults facing or going through and into puberty!

We are in the 21st Century, and still thousands, if not millions of women worldwide, are suffering and trying to cope with menopause, and the symptoms of this condition!

Puberty and menopause are both natural body processes that have been going on during our constant development as human beings and in earlier species. Had puberty and the later menopause not been a process of evolution, the human population of the world today would possibly not be in existence, so why then are these two subjects such taboo in many families, cultures, and groups?

Puberty is driven by the bodies sex hormones, mainly estrogen, in females, and testosterone in males. These hormones engage with the body's time clock to work and start the process of change from a child to adult. This process into maturity allows for survival of the species.

Menopause is driven in females by the body no longer needing the quantity of necessary hormones, mainly estrogen, to reproduce; therefore, the body and brain make the necessary adjustments to the sex hormones released! This reduction triggers the changes needed in the female body. Somewhat like puberty in many instances, the body takes on the change which can lead to different behaviours, and, in some instances, a person's difficulty to manage those changes!

So, what does happen and speaking as a teacher of psychology? Many hormones work in connection with and to the human brain; the brain needs to work in unison with the hormones and body clock, each is connected to the body's endocrine system. The endocrine system works with your body's electrical system. This electrical system is connected to your neuron pathways which run around your body; they make contact and deliver information, including some necessary hormones that allows your body to work.

If we are to look at the female menstrual cycle and the timing of the cycles, it will give you some idea of how each part of the body, hormones, brain, and electronics system is interconnected. It becomes difficult to stay healthy if either one or the other isn't working properly!

With menopause, the body is making its own adjustments, according to the body clock, through the electrical system and the quantity of sex hormones delivered or not delivered to the different parts of the female body. It's the adjustments in hormone delivery or non-delivery that causes females to experience many different experiences during menopause!

This is all very fine for me to write this information down, and as a teacher, and female, I have experienced the sudden changes to my body, brain, and physical non-wellbeing during what appeared at the time, to be a fast approach to, and through, menopause!

We know that every woman is different, and most women will experience menopause in different ways.

Many women do suffer in silence, their needs in all areas of life need to be met, this includes the workplace, home, including children, partners, and family members.

And, as said, each individual woman is so different in the way her body works, and each woman experiences the transition from being a fertile female to an infertile female is where this writing needs to go.

So many women love their womanhood, it is part of their femininity, their sexiness, and their lust for life. To wake up one day and feel confused or worthless and the knowledge of knowing that your confidence is diminishing is frightening and can be an overpowering emotional experience.

Not only is the female body changing, but also is the sense of worth, self-reliance and dignity. The assumption, *'it's only mum…!'* needs to stop.

Mums of the world communities are very

important. They bring to the home, workplace, community institutions such as hospitals, businesses, including the financial sectors, governments, education, and more, a wealth of experience, understanding and education, that without, many organisations, including governments, would find difficult to replace.

If we are to make a change to the existing Victorian attitude, we need to have many public conversations that not only include women, but governments, community groups and other high-profile organisations that have a loud community voice.

SO, WHAT IS PREMATURE MENOPAUSE?

As I now understand, though not an accepted title by many health practitioners, it's a female who enters the start of menopause before the age of fifty-one.

WHAT IS PERIMENOPAUSE?

From the information gathered, perimenopause means 'around the time,' or 'around menopause,' and refers to the time the body makes the natural transition to menopause. This transition may take a few months or up to ten years.

During this time, you may experience fluctuations in hot flushes, from being cool one minute to feeling overcome with experiencing a hot flush the next minute.

In perimenopause you may see different signs in irregular menstrual (period) cycles, these cycles may be longer or shorter. During your perimenopause, because of the changes in estrogen and progesterone levels, the ovulation time you had during your younger years, may not happen. Ovulation is when the mature egg, (ovum) is normally released from the ovary. Having said that, because you may experience spasmodic periods during this time, a female can still fall pregnant. Other signs may be vaginal dryness and itching of the vaginal area, the infamous 'hot flushes,' forgetfulness, headaches, and aching joints. With many of these conditions there are now treatments that may relieve some of the symptoms.

WHAT IS MENOPAUSE?
If you have not had a period for twelve months, then you are in menopause.

This natural ending is the sign that you are at the end of your reproductive life. It is the time when your ovaries no longer have the eggs, to release (ovum), into the fallopian tube.

During menopause, you may experience, difficulty sleeping (insomnia), night sweats, hot flushes, heart palpitations, vaginal irritation and dryness, urinary tract infections, mood changes, and mood swings; you may feel anxious, angry, upset, or feel you 'are on a short fuse', muscle and joint pain, being indecisive, and have low energy.

As I write the above and with a reflection on my own experiences of menopause, I recall, experiencing most of the above signs, but over just a few months. My recall of the experience of lying on the kitchen floor, as mentioned in Chapter Two, in absolute agony, while my husband looked on, is still a nightmare event in my life.

The pain went in spasms, close to that of labour contractions, at one of the pauses, I took some pain relief pills, but then the pain would start again. As the medication slowly took hold, the pain reduced, and eventually, I went back to bed. My head and body were in a whirlwind event, I could not think properly, let alone study, or work appropriately in my paid work! I was a total body and mind mess, and, at the time, I didn't know 'WHY?'

During the processes of change, an old friend

came back into my life. I would go for a coffee after work and not rush home to cook the evening meal as I always had done. I can remember the washing and ironing mounting up and, I didn't care!

The marriage had become just an existence! And yet, it was not what I wanted, but through times of change, we may start to re-evaluate the lifestyle we are living within! My husband and I didn't laugh, life had become serious, too serious for love to survive!

With the development of the friendship, I was learning to laugh again, and to enjoy just sitting and talking about nonsense content, it was a refreshing experience!

One night, I went out for a drink and had too much, this was within a few days after the episode of pain I experienced on the kitchen floor! I went to the bathroom, and there saw, what resembled a miscarriage in blood loss. It couldn't be that, as my fallopian tubes were tied, (tubal ligation), and, as a married woman, I had not had intercourse for several months. After the in-depth reading done for this book, I now believe, if it wasn't the leftover eggs, expelling themselves from the ovaries, was it the mucus lining of the uterus? I may never know the answer! I do know now it was my body's own mechanism of extraction that allowed my body to either eject or flush out any unneeded waste that may eventually cause sickness or discomfort!

The experience my body went through that night in the bathroom was so completely different to any other experience I had experienced with the menstrual cycle. The natural dilation of the vagina to allow the eggs or body waste to release, was, not painful, but the extraction was frightening when seeing the volume of blood loss in the toilet pan!

The period experienced that night was the last period and none have happened since.

Over this time, I was trying to hold everything together! When a woman sees herself as 'a cog in the wheel,' and that is all; the cog, simply, keeps the home running smoothly and adjustments aren't modified, she just keeps within boundaries to keep everything running effortlessly, cracks will appear in the marriage. Having a different person to speak with and in my life, was not an accepted part of traditional marriage, in what was, I see now as an outdated attitude. So many wrongs can be righted, if we only take the time to sit and talk things through…!

It has taken many years to speak about my experience with menopause, and it wasn't easy to do, but I'm glad the words are now down on paper because there may be other women experiencing similar body changes, especially as the world has experienced the Covid pandemic, and it is still too early to see the outcomes or residue related to the virus and women's health. I hope my story helps in some way.

SO, WHAT IS POST-MENOPAUSE?
For some women, the hot flushes may reduce or become a 'thing of the past', vaginal dryness may still exist, if you are worried, please see a health practitioner or doctor.

Weight gain is possibly one of the biggest changes for many women. As the author of the book, *'Devils In Our Food',* this is one of my 'war cries', **'do not eat processed, trans fat or molecule manipulated foods of any type!'** Weight after menopause can increase quickly. Eat a healthy diet of whole foods, whole grains, nuts, fruit, and other foods that are naturally grown and produced.

If you are post-menopausal, regular exercise is of great importance. Despite the glitzy advertising by fast food chains, showing the older population eating fast food, do not be enticed to eat junk food. Keep to a healthy diet of fresh food and vegetables, after all, you want to keep your body, brain, and hormones in good order!

OVER THE LAST THIRTY YEARS

It is only recently that I had a CAT scan and discovered that the left ovary no longer exists! During the research for this book, I have also discovered that ovaries do die. My only assumption can be, was the episode on the kitchen floor so many years ago, was in fact, the ovary dying, and it was in the last lease of its life! At least, I now know some of the causes for the chronic pain, and the madness of my behaviour, over the time and while experiencing perimenopause!

I have spoken to many post-menopausal women over the last thirty years, many don't want broken marriages, but they do want to see changes happen in the human attitude towards women's menopause and how it is perceived in the adult population.

PREMATURE MENOPAUSE YOU KNOW...!

Yes, I'm still on the go, *'premature menopause...'* I've been told, and I'm unable to know...!

Still a mountain of work to do before I can go...

'Take some rest', they say, regardless, I still cannot stop, and still, I must grow...!

I want to know much more for nature has me in store...!

Some hot sweats I've been told, and had them last night, woke up in a fright...!

Goodness, the bed was a wet mess, and yet the body had more...,
not to mention, some headaches my head had in store...!

No, premature menopause they say, *'should not have symptoms', and it's just a stage, regardless of age...!*

Premature menopause, I'm waiting for the next event, couldn't think of anything nicer than sleeping in the tent...

Air flow I need, and just for the breeze, *'there's still more to come,'* they emphasise and yet...

I've had enough, and am only partway through...

A life changing event, and Oh...,

This body adjusting....!

There's nothing to do, but go on the journey to what happens next, and living it through...!

PREMATURE MENOPAUSE YOU KNOW...!

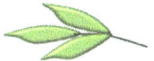

See menopause as a positive time; a time of thinking and doing the things you have been waiting to do. Hobbies are a great way forward. Writing these books, though a lot of hard work, I have been waiting to do since I was seven years old, and this time allows me to follow my dream.

Christine

As a mature woman, we can look on, and observe...

We can look at the journey our younger people are on...

Sometimes, we want to reach out, but if we do this, our young will not learn and grow...

Learning to observe is part of the richness and fabric of this later age – there's no time to think about the 'what if's' – they are gone and far away...!

You are now on your pathway, seeking, learning, growing, and gaining knowledge for your own wellbeing of mind heart and soul...!

CHAPTER FIVE
STILL WANTING TO KNOW MORE...

I continue to research and as I trawl through so much information, I had to ask myself, am I looking at this subject from the wrong angle or wrong end?

I have collected case studies, but nothing had prepared me for the facts, that women's suicide rates in the United Kingdom, between the ages of forty-five to fifty-four had indeed increased by six percent in 2021.[5]

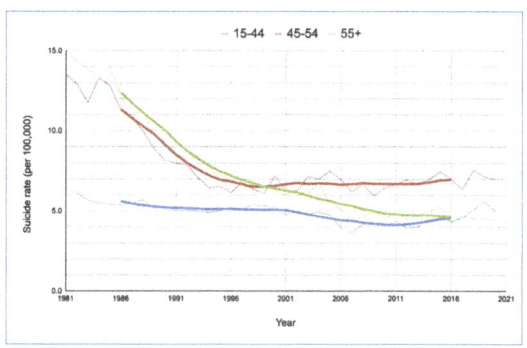

Image courtesy ITV News

---

[5] [4] Office of National Statistics (ONS) UK. 17th November 2021 *physical, emotional, and psychological symptoms that can be challenging to deal with.*

Dee Murray, CEO of the 'Menopause Experts Group' says, *"Menopause affects every woman differently, but for many it can bring unpleasant mental health issues like depression, anxiety and stress are hard to deal with, and many women will not know that they can commonly be caused by menopause. We cannot ignore what is happening or let these women suffer.*

"Women who are not aware they are going through menopause can be caught off guard by feelings of worthlessness, confusion, and a complete lack of confidence."

For the information I was looking for, though there have been great breakthroughs in research and menopause research; it is the vast scope of differences within each of us that makes this a difficult subject to, not only speak about, but to isolate a single remedy or diagnosis!

PERIMENOPAUSAL DEPRESSION – AN UNDER RECOGNISED ENTITY

In research carried out by Professor Jayashri Kulkarni, *"Mental health disorders can have devastating impacts on women as they approach menopause. This phase of a woman's life, typically between 42 and 52 years of age, is known as the 'perimenopause' and mental illness is very prevalent, in women at this stage. The risk of serious depression is significantly increased in perimenopausal women. The adverse impact also affects her family and society.*

Research specifically targeting the mental health of perimenopausal women is lacking. There is a gap in the recognition and provision of appropriate treatments for middle-aged women experiencing depression related to the hormonal changes of the menopause."[6]

In another article, Rebecca Joy Stanborough,

---

[6] https://www.nps.org.au/ - Australian Prescriber

(Healthline), has identified some key areas that affect women's health, during perimenopause, these being:

- allergies
- anxiety
- bloating
- breast pain and tenderness
- burning tongue
- hair loss
- heart palpitations
- hormonal headache
- hot flushes
- irregular periods
- irritability
- itchy skin
- joint pain
- lack of concentration
- low libido
- memory loss
- mood swings
- muscle tension
- night sweats

- osteoporosis
- panic disorder
- sleep disorders
- tingling extremities
- vaginal dryness
- weight gain[7]

All of which, from my research, indicate that the above is the work of our changing hormones.

THE STORY CONTINUES

Now, having done in-depth reading and further research into the way our hormones can work in different ways and on different body clocks, it does start to give some answers.

Having said that, though I was diagnosed as being in premature menopause, and as my research reveals, which I now believe to be perimenopause. Further research reveals, *'there should be no symptoms with pre-menopause…!'*

---

[7] Rebecca Joy Stanborough, MFA (healthline.com)

For many women, being diagnosed as pre-menopausal, there is a reason for going to the doctor if they have a concern about their health; this was the reason I had taken a trip to the doctor…!

When diagnosed, I can remember experiencing a few hot night sweats, but it wasn't every night, nor was it over a long period of time. Now with insight, the perimenopause came with a bang, possibly more a tsunami in my real-life experiences.

Continuing with my research, a female can experience menopause, and as said, in her twenties and there may be many reasons for this:

- Stress
- Smoking
- Exposure to toxins
- Ovarian surgery
- Viral infections and diseases
- Genetic differences

- Autoimmune disorders and
- Low estrogen supplies to the body.

I now believe that my own menopause was brought on by the glandular fever virus as, I too, as the doctor explained, '...*you are one of three other women diagnosed at this time with glandular fever and are pre-menopausal...!*'

Whilst, through undertaking strenuous research, the hormones that supply the female body with the necessary hormones to keep the womanly parts functioning, it comes as no surprise that our hormone supply can be interrupted by any of the previously spoken about experiences. Hormones, like so many parts of the human system are susceptible to changes brought on by virus attack, shock, or the changes in life we may experience.

When the body goes into shock, either male or female, the balanced systems within the body, alter and may change permanently. It is not only the bodily system but the many systems that are operated through and via the body's brain.

Though there are many hormones working in the body, such as insulin, gonadotropin, adrenaline and more, many work from within, not only the brain, and some work in conjunction with other hormones!

In writing my book *'Hormones, Puberty & Your Child'*, I speak about the many areas of abuse that so many children go through in their daily lives, apart from it being shocking, it should not happen. Severe experiences can and do alter our lives and our life direction. Here are the areas we have identified that many of the children go through in this 21st Century: bombardment from social media, vaping at school or witnessing vaping, underage sexual activities, drugs and drug exposure, peer pressure, bullying, depression, unwanted pregnancies, lack of confidence, self-harm, underage drinking, sexually transmitted diseases (STD) and in some instances, criminal acts. The previously spoken about events in younger people's lives may also happen as we get older. When the senses, then the brain which contains the memory, goes through any shock or like any of the above disturbances, it will alter the neuron network of the brain, which may interfere with the regular hormone supply to the body and disrupt the hormone messaging to and from the brain.

Each person, child, or adult will take in information in a different way, that altered information may change the way we each manage the same received information!

A young woman experiencing premature menopause, or menopause may have had experiences, that have indeed, disrupted her regular hormone supply and that brings into her life a 'life changing' event. However, when changes happen, each female experiencing such changes needs love and understanding during the process of change.

It is not only the supply of estrogen that can be interrupted, but also the supply of other essential hormones through the processes of change. When the estrogen level is low, and under normal conditions, another hormone can and may 'kick in' to help the estrogen supply level to come to the accepted level that allows the body to function and work properly. When the body's clock is interrupted through abuse or negative experiences, the communication between the brain and the needed hormones, may also become disengaged!

If a female is wondering why there are changes happening to her body, she may be in menopause; here are some signs to look for:

VAGINAL WELLBEING
As the reading and research continues, it's interesting to learn about vaginal dryness and how vulvovaginal atrophy[8] or (VVA) may progress as

---
Atrophy is when a body part or organ has a reduction in size or reduction in cells.

we go through certain life stages. Through the reduction of estrogen, the vaginal track also undergoes its different stages of wellbeing. Thus, the reduction of the estrogen hormone, the vaginal flora is also reducing leading to dryness, soreness, and itching. The natural flora of the vagina is changing!

SOME AGE GUIDELINES

We know that every woman is different and there is not one linear approach that fits all females. Following is an age schema that may assist with keeping in mind how your hormones are functioning:

Ages 40 to 45

"*A couple of missed periods when you're 40 might lead you to think you're pregnant, but it's also possible to begin menopause around this age. About 5 percent of women go into early menopause, experiencing symptoms between the ages of 40 and 45. One percent of women go into premature menopause before age 40.*

Signs you're in early menopause include:
- *missing more than three periods in a row*
- *heavier or lighter than usual periods*
- *trouble sleeping*
- *weight gain*
- *hot flushes*
- *vaginal dryness.*

Ages 45 to 50

"Many biological females enter the perimenopausal phase in their late 40s. Perimenopause means "around menopause."

At this stage, your estrogen and progesterone production slow, and you begin to make the transition into menopause.

"Perimenopause can last 7-14 years. You'll likely still get a period during this time, but your menstrual cycles will become more erratic.

Symptoms of perimenopause are due to rising and falling estrogen levels in your body. You may experience:

- *hot flushes*
- *mood swings*
- *night sweats*
- *vaginal dryness*
- *difficulty sleeping*
- *changes in sex drive*
- *trouble concentrating*
- *hair loss*
- *fast heart rate*
- *urinary problems.*

Ages 50 to 55

"During your early 50s, you may be in menopause, or you may be making the final transition into this phase. At this point, your ovaries are no longer releasing eggs or making much estrogen.

Ages 60 to 65

"A small percentage of Assigned Females At Birth, (AFAB) folks are late going into menopause. This

isn't necessarily a bad thing. Studies of late menopause show a lower risk of:
- *heart attack*
- *stroke*
- *osteoporosis*

It's also linked to a longer life expectancy. Researchers believe that prolonged exposure to estrogen protects the heart and bones."[9]

Article: Stephanie Watson

SUMMING UP

Of this chapter, it is the movement of hormones within the female body and brain, life experiences, genetic profile, lifestyle, and the internal female's body clock that organises how hormones work, when they start, as in puberty onset, or when the finish is menopause!

We can try to make some changes, but like the Covid pandemic, hormones are unpredictable and will work to their own variables. As the owners of

---

[9] Symptoms of Menopause at Every Age: 40 to 65 (healthline.com)

the hormones, we can monitor, watch for, and try to recognise the subtle changes that take place in our body and brain, stay alert and not be of the assumption, that because we don't see them, they are not working; hormones are our responsibility and as I say to the children, *'when hormones perform, you perform…!'* It helps hormone health by having a continuous, healthy sustainable diet.

STILL WANT TO KNOW MORE...?

Evasive they seem to be, but they are there and working, though you can't see....

We each have these miniscule chemicals working, but a healthy diet might just be the key...!

At times they do the untold, like becoming less as we age and want to be free...

Many women have suffered through the years without ever knowing, it was the hormones that caused the night sweats and the foregoing...!

As a child, we were not aware, that growing would lead us right there....

Now, we know, and our parents experienced some of the same, but got on without, and no one to blame...!

You see, it has happened for generations past, our grandmothers and great grandmothers endured the challenges, that made them last...

The hormones who work and sometimes get tired, will continue to work, and do their best, but like us all, they sometimes need time out, and time to take a rest...!

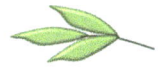

The journey we go through is nothing new and for thousands of years our grandmothers and great grandmothers have all experienced the many experiences we experience in the 21st Century...!

Having said that, we have little said from those wise ladies of our past – they travelled their journey and did not complain, but those days are long-ago...!

We now need to consider our future females and the knowledge we can give to them; it is now our responsibility to let them know the story of menopause...

CHAPTER SIX
CASE STUDIES – THE REALITY!

Throughout this book, I have spoken of eating a healthy diet. By understanding, that hormones, to work effectively, also need to have healthy molecules fed to them.

If the food and drink we consume has not got the quality of goodness that our body needs, we can expect to become sick. Hormones are no different to any other part of the human body or brain, like that expensive car, you would not put rubbish petrol in its tank, so why would you put rubbish food in your stomach, (your tank)? You simply will not work properly if you don't have good fuel in your tank….!

Of course, there are many contributing factors to having healthy hormones, but your diet will possibly dictate how your hormones work!

Hormones and the endocrine system are just part

of the story to running an efficient body. You will now understand, the body has many different and interconnecting systems; each system works effectively when all the systems are working in harmony.

Sarah Sandison,[10] (Liverpool Echo)

SHORT EXTRACTS – CASE STUDIES

Laura adds: *"These hot flushes! I used to be nice and now it's like I wake up and choose violence."*

Jenni adds: *"I'm in perimenopause and honestly, I've never felt so unattractive in my whole entire life. If my partner was to cheat on me whilst I'm struggling, it would destroy me!"*

Clare says: *"I'm deep in perimenopause at the moment and it's hit me hard, mentally and physically. It also riddles me with anxiety that my other half will get fed up of my lower sex drive. I*

---

[10] https://www.liverpoolecho.co.uk

don't think he would cheat or leave, but the fear is there."

Sam adds: *"I've got this all going on right now! Just been prescribed testosterone to see if it helps. Luckily, I have a lovely fella who gets it."*

Deb says: *"I was diagnosed with early menopause two years ago at 40 and it has been a living hell, to be honest. But I feel like I'm coming out the other side now. HRT and collagen supplements are the one! Nobody in the medical profession listens to you, or how you are feeling, I'm lucky I have the nicest and most amazing husband in the world. Start taking collagen now, get all the bone broth in you that you can, it really helps! Apple cider vinegar is fantastic too. Don't dread it, it's actually quite liberating, once you stop wanting to stab everything and everyone!"*

Meg Matthews has been very open about her first and unexpected symptoms of menopause. In a recent interview for Planet Mindful she revealed: *"My symptoms were all linked to mental health."* She added: *"I had lots of anxiety, lots of overwhelming feelings towards life and I became agoraphobic. I didn't leave the house for three months and my world became smaller and smaller."*

Sarah continues with her article: *"It's not just women who need to be aware of the signs and symptoms of menopause. Men need to be able to look out for them and spot them in the women around them."*

In the sadness of the research, Sarah continues, *"…widower David Salmon is calling for people to understand more about the symptoms of menopause. David's is a hard-hitting story, of a husband who lost his wife to suicide during the menopause. His wife Linda took her own life after struggling with what doctors called 'treatment resistant depression'. Mr. Salmon had no idea that menopause caused anxiety and suicidal thoughts until he was watching a BBC television program, that included information about how suddenly and severely mental health can deteriorate during perimenopause and menopause.*

David worked closely with campaigners GenM[11] to tell his story as part of their efforts to raise awareness amongst men, of the menopause and its symptoms."

Sam, while I was interviewing her for this book, said, *"I don't know about pre-menopausal, but I can tell you, perimenopause was far worse than I could have imagined. I thought I would treat the condition with traditional therapies; I was living in Asia then, so I tried tofu, it didn't work for me, so I went straight back to the doctor; he had suggested HRT treatment previously! Within a couple of weeks, after starting with HRT, I was feeling so much better...!"*

---

[11] GenM | The Menopause Partner for Brands (gen-m.com)

Florence, says, *"I stayed on HRT until I was in my sixties, it was all working OK, but then, I thought I would let nature take its course…!"* Florence raises her eyes skywards, then takes a deep breath, and says, *"Oh boy,' then did I know it…? I'm OK now but I didn't realise what I would go through once stopping the HRT treatment…!"*

My own story has left me completely dumbfounded, I behaved in a way that was completely out of character and, even as a teenager, I would never have done the things I did when I was in perimenopause. I went out, had too much to drink, and not a care in the world. I was completely blind to my responsibilities and my family. I'm not proud of my behaviour, but it does go back to how we are treated as a woman in our relationship.

So many women can carry anger over past events, and one day, if not rectified, that anger will surface.

Sue said, *"I broke up with my husband, and I'm not proud, I didn't realise at the time, I was menopausal, but I had over twenty affairs, all short-term, but that is what I had to do, I couldn't stop myself!"*

Moving back to food quality and how, when the whole good food molecule is missing from our essential food intake, it can and may lead to devastating outcomes! It is not only our hormones that need nurturing and goodness but our whole and complete self, benefits from eating a good food diet!

In the following case study, though it may not be typical of a multiple sclerosis diagnosis, it will give you some idea of the importance of eating a healthy diet.

CASE STUDY
I once knew a man who insisted on eating every night and every day for every meal, fried chips,

fried eggs, and baked beans. His mother, bless her, could not change the menu. Twelve months a year and in all the years I knew him, he had the same diet.

Just recently there has been a scientific breakthrough into the causes of multiple sclerosis; sadly, this young man was diagnosed with this condition in his early twenties. The breakthrough relates to a lack of folic acid as being and part of the cause of this disease. Accordingly, this condition is known to cause damage to the autoimmune system through the breakdown of the myeline sheaf that surrounds the nerve fibres in the brain and spinal cord. There are no known causes for the condition, but it may come from genetic or by environmental influences, as in the food we eat.

Folic acid is vital to the body and brain's nerve wellbeing, and like so many natural foods, if folic acid is missing from the diet, then your body will let you know as you become unwell. Please always look at the food quality of the food you eat.

Sadly, the young man died in his late twenties. We may never know the exact cause of his illness, but the history of the study should ring alarm bells when it may be related to poor quality food eaten...!

CASE STUDY

In 2019, the following article was seen in The Telegraph, United Kingdom. The article is about '*a boy who only ate white bread, crisps, chips, and processed meat for about a decade. The seventeen-year-old, after eating this diet has now been classified as legally blind and deaf.*'[12]

Bad eating habits need to be broken early and before the person has the mental time to establish them.

---

[12] Dominic Lipinski/PA Lizzie Roberts, The Telegraph UK 3/9/2019

Hormones need healthy foods, foods such as rich leafy green vegetables, including cabbage, beans, nuts, fruits including lemons, melons, strawberries, bananas, and oranges; all are rich in folic acid.

In the 21st Century, many foods are contaminated through molecule manipulation, synthetic processing or through synthetic food additive colours being added to the ingredients. Little do people realise, that these so called, 'modern foods' may be the cause of many health problems, debilitating health conditions and other ailments within the human system and brain. If eaten in quantities, with limitation on natural food molecule intake, this may lead to many illnesses of the feeling or 'not feeling well!'

Your hormones work with your neuron messages sent from your brain to your limbs and other parts of your body, including your uterus and ovaries!

Brain starvation is also a consideration. When poor quality food is eaten, you may find it difficult to concentrate and have prolonged times of 'brain fog'. This condition limits concentration and gives you 'slow reaction' times in many jobs or hobbies you may want to pursue....

Persistent 'brain fog' is also your alarm bell that your body and brain may be experiencing a form of malnutrition brought on by eating poor quality food or drinking synthetic drinks with altered molecules and synthetic colouring!

When the body does not work, we do not work...!

Like so many parts of the human body and brain, the vagina needs to be healthy and have healthy bacteria. When the balance is disrupted as in the reduction of estrogen, then more sinister bacteria have the chance to grow and multiply. This multiplication of dangerous bacteria such as Gardnerella, Streptococcus, and Prevotella can lead to health problems and severe dryness of the vagina and painful experiences during intercourse. It can also lead to lower libido and sexual satisfaction.

Regardless of age, female health is heightened by the intake of a quality food diet, regular exercise, and the ability to think clearly and proactively, having regular rest and sleep, taking time out to enjoy the moments; each of these activities allows the female body to keep replenished their sexual health, and womanly parts!

WHAT ARE GOVERNMENTS DOING?
Female menopause is almost a forgotten topic. Our great grandmothers put up with it; many had shortened lives, our grandmothers, also put up with it, and our mothers! Now it is time for changes. A change in attitude is essential. A change in attitudes by most of the male population, this includes governments. A change in attitudes by employers and family members all

needs to happen in a hurry.

AUSTRALIAN GOVERNMENT

Whilst the Australian Government has a clause within its document, National Women's Health Strategy, 2020-2030, *"Menopause transition can affect women's physical and mental health and increases risk for future cardiometabolic health*.

This document outlines the governments approach over ten years; it does not outline necessary strategies that can be taken. In Principle 4 – A focus on prevention, it states, *"Shift from a purely medical model to a blended medical and psychosocial model, to consider an individual's social economic and cultural context to personalise health care."*

This relates to several different health conditions, not necessarily menopause which is a total condition experienced by all females.

UNITED KINGDOM GOVERNMENT

Press release, 2022: Nation unites to tackle menopause taskforce. Ministers and senior clinicians from across all 4 nations will come together today for the inaugural meeting of the UK Menopause Taskforce.

- First meeting of UK Menopause Taskforce to co- ordinate and work together on support for women across all nations.
- Consultation launched into reclassification of low-dose hormone replacement therapy (HRT) product Gina.

Formation of taskforce comes ahead of publication of first government-led Women's Health Strategy for England to tackle the gender health gap.

It does seem on the face of it, the UK, might be ahead of Australia in its proactive support of women and the menopausal debate.

A LAST UPLIFTING NOTE

Since my transition through menopause, I have

found that taking a teaspoonful of gelatine in a glass of fresh juice each day works to relieve skeletal discomfort in my groin area. Through this simple process, my health, energy, movement, and wellbeing have improved dramatically. When buying gelatine, buy, if you can, pure, unflavoured 225 bloom gelatine, or buy from a trusted source.

225 bloom is a high-grade product and is from grass fed, organic beef. It provides eight of the nine essential amino acids, not synthesized by the human body, but are essential to maintain good health.

Gelatine promotes gut and digestive health, helps to maintain, and stabilise appetite which assists with healthy eating habits and reduces food craving. It also helps with establishing weight control, assists with muscle recovery after exercise or injury; helps to develop strong bones, reduce pain and inflammation in joints; assists with hair and nail revitalisation, and assists in developing a healthy immune system.

Do not buy gelatine that has any preservative, colour, or artificial additives. Always look to see if the gelatine has additive numbers, if it does, do not buy; shop around to buy a safe product.

As age moves on, I've had my latest bone scan, rather than my bone density decreasing, it has gone up a bit. My doctor's comment, *'I don't know what you are doing, but keep doing it.'* I also take a regular supply of magnesium each day.

If you have concerns about your health, please seek professional medical advice.

HEALTHY FOOD, THE WHOLE FOOD MOLECULE IS NEEDED

It's the healthy food molecule that keeps us well; it helps our body repair and our brain in good condition, so can't you tell...?

If you eat food that's not fit for purpose, you will soon know more, for your stomach and brain you will not ignore...!

It's the greedy food producers that add to the mix, not good ingredients and its left up to us to remedy and fix...!

There are such very good foods to eat, some so good, you will know...
Because you can feel from your head to your toe...!

It's not much to ask of a body that's served, not to mention those hormones who want to do more, but how can they, if the fuel in the tank is contaminated and poor...!

There are quick solutions to feeling so ill, but it is far more advanced than taking a pill...!

Please look to your diet, to see how it works...!

If you want to know and want to energise

your 'GO'...

It's now time for your health to sew...!

As each woman is different, there is no 'one fix', but by reading extra and informative information, we can search to find what helps us to live through, what can be, a demanding and stressful time, in a woman's life. Together with taking the gelatine in a fruit juice drink, doing regular exercises, and staying mentally positive, each day, I have found that I can achieve so much more, more possibly than before I went through the stages of menopause!

Christine

THE GHOST OF FEMALE MENOPAUSE

We have just explored the Ghost of Female Menopause….

With so much information and far too much to be ignored…!

Women have suffered far too long, for now their turn to be heard out of the throng….!

Show respect we each need to know, for our bodies we give for each generation to grow…!

Now is the time to give her the space because we are fifty percent of the human race…!

Washing is done, ironing too, without any question and out of the blue…!

Now, for over three hundred thousand years and maybe much more, we have brought forward the children and life to restore…!

Children will continue to be born, and yet, we know that domestic violence exists….!

From the bodies of females, where the worlds' future babies will grow, we want re-assurance and for everyone to know…!

The knowledge is learnt, and change is now here…This cannot be ignored ….!

Attitudes are stubborn, but they need to change,
in fact, difficult to do...!

But attitudes must change, menopause will
continue, there's no turning back...!

It's the ghosts of the past and in the thinking, we
need to attack...!

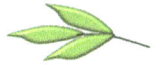

We have come a long way since the start of the journey; we can only learn from the experiences we have....!

Having said that, if we have the information and learning support needed, many women will find the journey of menopause an easier process.

As females, we cannot escape menopause, therefore we need to speak up, speak loudly so that the world knows, this is not a journey we should travel alone....!

YOUR NOTES

REFERENCES

Research, Dr. Helen O'Connell, Vincenzo, and Giulia Puppo Five things you should know about the clitoris (medicalnewstoday.com)

Office of National Statistics (ONS) UK. 17th November 2021

Dee Murray, CEO – 'Menopause Experts Group'

https://www.nps.org.au/ - Australian Prescriber

Rebecca Joy Stanborough – MFA (healthline.com)

Stephanie Watson – Symptoms of Menopause at Every Age: 40 to 65 (healthline.com)

Sarah Sanderson – https://www.liverpoolecho.co.uk

GenM The Menopause Partner for Brands (gen-m.com)

Dominic Lipinski/PA Lizzie Roberts, The Telegraph UK 3/9/2019

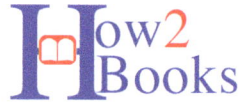

See our website: www.how2books.com.au

ISBN:978-0-6457284-4-6

www.ingramcontent.com/pod-product-compliance
Lightning Source LLC
Chambersburg PA
CBHW051538010526
44107CB00064B/2771